Longevity Nutrition Blueprint

Advanced Fasting, Protein Cycling, and Micronutrient Strategies for Lifelong Health

By Joe Correa

Published by Live Stronger Faster

This book is for educational and informational purposes only. The author and publisher are not engaged in rendering legal, financial, or other professional advice. Readers should consult a qualified professional before making any financial decisions.

First Edition

Table of Contents

Introduction 5

Chapter 1: Nutrition as a Biological Signal, Not a Calorie Equation........ 11

Chapter 2: Metabolic Flexibility: Teaching the Body to Switch, Not Struggle........ 18

Chapter 3: Advanced Fasting Windows: Timing Autophagy Without Breaking the System........ 25

Chapter 4: Protein Cycling for Longevity: Building Without Accelerating Aging........ 31

Chapter 5: Micronutrient Precision: Feeding the Enzymes That Control Aging........ 37

Chapter 6: Nutrient Density & Food Diversity: Designing a Longevity Plate........ 44

Chapter 7: Carbohydrate Cycling for Longevity: Fueling Performance Without Accelerating Aging........ 50

Chapter 8: Circadian Nutrition: Aligning Meals With the Body's Longevity Clock........ 57

Chapter 9: Weekly & Seasonal Nutrition Cycles: Reintroducing Biological Contrast Across Time........ 64

Chapter 10: Integrating the Longevity Nutrition System: Designing a Lifelong Blueprint........ 71

Chapter 11: Adaptive Nutrition Across the Lifespan: Evolving Longevity From Youth to Late Life..78

Epilogue..85

Introduction

Longevity is not created by a single food, a single supplement, or a single dietary philosophy. It is constructed through **nutritional signaling**—the precise, repeated messages sent to your cells every day through calories, macronutrients, micronutrients, timing, and metabolic stress. Food is not merely fuel; it is instruction. Every meal either accelerates aging or slows it, either inflames systems or restores them, either programs resilience or invites breakdown. This book exists to correct the most damaging misconception in modern health: that eating for longevity is simply about eating "healthy foods." Longevity nutrition is about **eating intelligently, cyclically, strategically, and intentionally across time**.

In the earlier books of this series, you learned how aging unfolds at the cellular, mitochondrial, hormonal, inflammatory, and epigenetic levels. You now understand that lifespan and healthspan are shaped by autophagy, mitochondrial efficiency, insulin signaling, inflammation control, and gene expression. Nutrition touches every one of these systems simultaneously. It is the master lever that can either amplify the benefits of those systems—or completely override them. This is why populations with access to the best supplements, advanced medical care, and exercise technology can still age rapidly if their nutrition sends the wrong biological signals. Longevity nutrition is not static; it is **adaptive, rhythmic, and personalized**.

The Longevity Nutrition Blueprint introduces three advanced pillars that separate anti-aging science from conventional dieting: **fasting intelligence, protein cycling, and micronutrient precision**. These strategies are not trends. They are rooted in evolutionary biology, clinical research, and long-lived population data. When combined correctly, they create an internal environment where cellular repair outpaces cellular damage, where metabolic flexibility replaces metabolic fragility, and where nutrient sufficiency exists without excess. This is the difference between merely surviving longer and remaining biologically youthful while doing so.

Fasting, when misunderstood, becomes stress. When applied strategically, it becomes **one of the most powerful longevity tools available to humans**. This book will dismantle the myth that longer fasts are always better or that fasting is only about calorie reduction. Instead, you will learn how different fasting windows activate distinct repair pathways, how fasting interacts with hormones differently at various life stages, and how improper fasting can sabotage longevity by elevating cortisol, suppressing thyroid function, or accelerating muscle loss. Longevity fasting is not starvation—it is **metabolic choreography**, designed to stimulate autophagy without breaking resilience.

Protein is the most misunderstood macronutrient in longevity science. On one side, low-protein advocates point to reduced mTOR signaling and lifespan extension. On the other, high-protein proponents emphasize muscle preservation, metabolic health, and functional aging. Both sides are partially correct—and incomplete. Longevity does not demand chronic protein restriction or chronic protein excess. It demands **protein cycling**. In this book, you will learn how to strategically alternate between periods of higher protein intake for tissue repair and muscle preservation, and lower protein phases that promote autophagy, insulin sensitivity, and cellular cleanup. Protein cycling allows you to gain the benefits of growth without paying the biological cost of constant growth signaling.

Micronutrients are often treated as an afterthought, yet they determine whether every other longevity strategy succeeds or fails. Deficiencies in magnesium, zinc, selenium, iodine, B vitamins, and fat-soluble nutrients silently accelerate aging by impairing mitochondrial enzymes, hormone synthesis, detoxification pathways, and DNA repair. At the same time, excessive supplementation can disrupt nutrient balance and create new problems. The Longevity Nutrition Blueprint teaches **micronutrient sufficiency without overload**, showing you how to meet biological needs through food-first strategies, targeted supplementation, and seasonal adjustment. Longevity nutrition is about balance—not minimalism and not excess.

One of the most dangerous ideas in modern nutrition is the belief that the same diet should be followed every day for years. Biological systems thrive on **variation**, not monotony. The human body evolved in an environment of feast and famine, nutrient abundance and scarcity, protein surges and protein gaps. When nutrition becomes repetitive, signaling becomes distorted. This book introduces the concept of **nutritional periodization for longevity**, where fasting cycles, protein intake, carbohydrate exposure, and micronutrient density shift intentionally across weeks, months, and seasons to maintain metabolic flexibility and cellular responsiveness.

Longevity nutrition must also be contextual. Age, sex, hormonal status, activity level, stress load, and sleep quality all determine how food is processed and how signals are interpreted. A fasting protocol that rejuvenates one person may deplete another. A protein intake that preserves muscle in midlife may accelerate aging if applied incorrectly later. This book will teach you how to **adjust nutritional strategy as**

biology changes, rather than rigidly clinging to one identity-based diet. Longevity belongs to those who adapt. Importantly, longevity nutrition is not about perfection. Chronic restriction, obsessive tracking, and fear-based eating increase stress hormones, disrupt sleep, and undermine immune resilience—ironically accelerating aging. The goal of this blueprint is **sustainable biological optimization**, not dietary extremism. You will learn how to build nutrition patterns that support long-term consistency, social flexibility, and psychological ease while still activating longevity pathways. A stressed, rigid body does not live longer—even if it eats "clean."

Throughout this book, nutrition will be reframed as a **systems-level intervention**. Fasting will be linked to autophagy, insulin sensitivity, and inflammation control. Protein cycling will be tied to muscle preservation, hormone balance, and mitochondrial efficiency. Micronutrients will be mapped to enzymatic repair, detoxification, and genetic stability. You will not be given meal plans to blindly follow. Instead, you will be taught **how to think like a longevity biologist**, enabling you to adjust food choices intelligently across life phases, goals, and conditions.

By the end of this book, you will understand why longevity nutrition cannot be reduced to calories alone, why timing often matters more than quantity, why cycles outperform constants, and why nourishment—not restriction—is the true foundation of extended healthspan. You will know how to use fasting without breaking your metabolism, protein without accelerating aging, and micronutrients without imbalance. Most importantly, you will understand how nutrition communicates with your biology—and how to ensure the message it sends is one of repair, resilience, and renewal.

Longevity is not accidental. It is engineered daily. This book is your blueprint.

Chapter 1

Nutrition as a Biological Signal, Not a Calorie Equation

Modern nutrition has been reduced to arithmetic. Calories in versus calories out. Macronutrient ratios. Portion sizes. Daily targets. While these metrics are useful for short-term weight manipulation, they fail entirely at explaining aging. The human body does not age because it consumed too many calories. It ages because it receives the wrong biological signals repeatedly over time. Nutrition is not a math problem. It is a communication system. Every bite of food delivers information that influences hormones, gene expression, cellular repair, inflammation, mitochondrial output, and nervous system tone. Longevity nutrition begins when food is understood as instruction rather than fuel.

When food enters the body, it does far more than provide energy. It activates pathways that tell cells whether to grow, repair, defend, or shut down. Glucose availability affects insulin signaling and inflammatory tone. Amino acids activate mTOR and protein synthesis pathways. Fatty acids influence membrane fluidity and hormone production. Micronutrients act as cofactors for thousands of enzymatic reactions that govern DNA repair, detoxification, and mitochondrial efficiency. Aging accelerates when these signals are chronically mismatched with the body's adaptive capacity. Longevity emerges when signals are timed, cycled, and balanced to favor repair over damage.

One of the most damaging nutritional myths is the belief that consistency means eating the same way every day. Biological systems are not designed for sameness. They are designed for variability. Throughout human evolution, food availability fluctuated. Periods of abundance were followed by scarcity. Protein intake rose and fell. Micronutrients varied seasonally. This variability trained cells to remain flexible, resilient, and responsive. When modern diets eliminate variability, cells become metabolically rigid. Insulin sensitivity declines. Autophagy slows. Inflammation rises. Longevity nutrition restores variability intentionally.

Fasting is the most obvious example of nutritional signaling. When food intake pauses, insulin drops, glucagon rises, and autophagy activates. Cells begin recycling damaged components, clearing misfolded proteins, and repairing DNA. However, fasting is not universally beneficial in all forms. Excessive fasting without adequate refeeding creates stress, suppresses thyroid output, elevates cortisol, and accelerates muscle loss. Longevity fasting is not about endurance or willpower. It is about selecting fasting windows that stimulate repair while preserving metabolic stability. This requires understanding context, not following trends.

Protein represents another critical signal. Protein intake tells the body whether it is time to build or conserve. High protein stimulates muscle growth, tissue repair, and immune resilience, but also increases mTOR signaling, which accelerates aging when chronically elevated. Low protein reduces growth signaling and enhances autophagy, but prolonged restriction leads to sarcopenia, frailty, and metabolic decline. Longevity does not demand choosing one side. It requires cycling between them. Protein cycling allows the body to experience growth and repair phases without paying the long-term cost of constant stimulation.

Micronutrients operate quietly but decisively. They do not provide calories, yet without them, energy production collapses. Magnesium stabilizes ATP. Zinc supports immune function and DNA repair. Selenium protects mitochondria from oxidative damage. Iodine enables thyroid hormone production. B vitamins drive methylation and neurotransmitter synthesis. Deficiencies create silent aging long before symptoms appear. At the same time, excessive supplementation disrupts balance and interferes with absorption. Longevity nutrition prioritizes sufficiency through food diversity and strategic support rather than megadosing.

Another overlooked factor in longevity nutrition is timing. The same meal eaten at different times produces different hormonal and metabolic outcomes. Eating late at night disrupts circadian rhythms, impairs glucose control, and suppresses melatonin. Front-loading nutrition earlier in the day improves insulin sensitivity and mitochondrial efficiency. Fasting aligned with circadian biology amplifies repair. Longevity nutrition integrates timing as a biological variable, not an afterthought.

Stress determines how nutrition is interpreted. A nutrient-dense meal consumed under chronic stress may produce inflammation rather than nourishment. Elevated cortisol alters digestion, impairs nutrient absorption, and shifts metabolism toward fat storage. Longevity nutrition cannot be separated from nervous system regulation. A calm system extracts benefit. A stressed system accelerates aging. This is why rigid diets often fail long-term. They increase psychological stress even as they attempt biological optimization.

Ultimately, longevity nutrition is about creating an internal environment where repair consistently exceeds damage. This does not require perfection. It requires pattern recognition. Repeated signals of abundance without scarcity accelerate aging. Repeated scarcity without nourishment weakens resilience. Longevity exists in oscillation. In learning how to alternate feeding and fasting, protein abundance and restraint, micronutrient density and metabolic rest, the body regains its adaptive intelligence. Nutrition becomes a tool for longevity rather than a source of confusion.

This chapter establishes the foundation for the Longevity Nutrition Blueprint. Before protocols, before schedules, before supplements, the mindset must shift. Food is not simply something to control. It is something to communicate with. When that communication becomes intentional, aging slows not because calories drop, but because biology listens.

The Signals That Changed Everything

At forty-six, Daniel believed he was doing everything right. He tracked calories meticulously, hit his protein goals daily, avoided sugar, exercised five times a week, and followed every rule he had been taught. Yet he felt older each year. His recovery slowed. His sleep fragmented. His energy dipped by midafternoon. Blood work showed rising inflammation markers and declining testosterone. Doctors told him it was normal aging. Daniel accepted the explanation reluctantly, assuming discipline was no longer enough.

What Daniel didn't realize was that his discipline had become biological noise. Every day looked the same. Every meal arrived at the same time. Every macronutrient ratio was identical. His body no longer received contrast. There were no repair signals, no metabolic challenges, no cellular pauses. Growth pathways remained activated continuously. Inflammation never fully resolved. His cells had become efficient at survival but terrible at renewal.

The shift began not with a new diet, but with a new question. Instead of asking how much he should eat, Daniel asked what message his food was sending. He learned that his constant protein intake kept mTOR elevated. His late-night meals disrupted circadian repair. His fear of fasting prevented autophagy from ever fully activating. For the first time, nutrition felt less like control and more like conversation.

Daniel began slowly. He introduced two fasting days per week, not as deprivation, but as recovery windows. He cycled protein intake, eating more on training days and less on rest days. He focused on micronutrient density instead of supplement stacks, adding seafood, leafy greens, nuts, and mineral-rich foods. He shifted his largest meal earlier in the day and allowed his evenings to quiet.

Within weeks, subtle changes appeared. Sleep deepened. Morning energy stabilized. Joint stiffness faded. Blood markers improved without weight loss being the primary goal.

Months later, muscle mass increased even with fewer calories overall. His body responded not because he ate less, but because it finally received varied, meaningful signals.

Daniel realized that aging had not been inevitable. It had been instructed. His old habits had unknowingly told his body to grow endlessly without repair, to stay fed without resting, to perform without restoring. By changing the signals, he changed the outcome. Nutrition became adaptive rather than rigid. Sustainable rather than exhausting.

The most powerful moment came when Daniel stopped fearing food and stopped fearing hunger. He trusted his biology again. Meals felt purposeful. Fasting felt restorative. Eating became aligned with seasons, stress levels, and activity rather than rules. His body regained intelligence it had lost under constant stimulation.

Daniel's story is not unique. It is repeated in every person who shifts from calorie control to biological signaling. Longevity does not arrive through restriction alone. It arrives when the body is reminded how to repair itself. Nutrition, when used intelligently, becomes the language through which youth is preserved—not forced, but invited.

This is the foundation of the Longevity Nutrition Blueprint. Not a diet to follow, but a system to understand. Not a rulebook, but a conversation with biology. Aging listens. And when spoken to correctly, it slows.

Chapter 2

Metabolic Flexibility: Teaching the Body to Switch, Not Struggle

Longevity is not determined by how efficiently the body uses one fuel source. It is determined by how easily it can switch between them. This ability, known as metabolic flexibility, defines whether the body adapts smoothly to stress or deteriorates under it. A metabolically flexible system transitions effortlessly between glucose and fat, between fed and fasted states, between energy expenditure and repair. A metabolically rigid system resists change, accumulates damage, and accelerates aging. Nutrition plays the primary role in teaching the body which state to prioritize—and how often to change.

In a healthy organism, metabolic flexibility is natural. After eating, insulin rises, glucose is used efficiently, and excess energy is stored appropriately. During fasting or energy demand, insulin falls, fat oxidation increases, and stored energy is released without stress. Aging begins when this switch becomes impaired. Chronically elevated insulin prevents fat mobilization. Frequent feeding suppresses metabolic rest. Constant carbohydrate availability removes the need for adaptation. Over time, the body forgets how to transition, and every metabolic shift becomes a struggle rather than a response.

Modern diets unintentionally train metabolic inflexibility. Continuous snacking, high glycemic foods, and fear of hunger keep insulin elevated throughout the day. The body remains locked in glucose dependency, unable to access fat stores efficiently. This creates energy volatility, inflammation, and mitochondrial overload. Longevity nutrition reverses this process by intentionally reintroducing metabolic contrast. Periods of feeding are followed by periods of rest. Carbohydrate availability fluctuates. Fat oxidation is reactivated. Flexibility is restored through experience, not force.

Fasting is one of the most effective tools for rebuilding metabolic flexibility when applied intelligently. Short fasting windows reduce insulin, activate fat oxidation, and improve mitochondrial efficiency. Longer fasting intervals deepen autophagy and increase cellular cleanup. However, fasting without metabolic readiness produces stress rather than adaptation. Individuals with poor mitochondrial function, thyroid dysregulation, or chronic cortisol elevation may require gradual exposure. Longevity fasting respects biological readiness rather than imposing uniform protocols.

Carbohydrates are often blamed for metabolic dysfunction, but the issue is not carbohydrates themselves—it is the absence of cycling. Carbohydrates serve essential functions in thyroid hormone conversion, serotonin production, and high-intensity performance. Eliminating them completely reduces metabolic adaptability rather than improving it. Longevity nutrition introduces carbohydrate cycling, where intake increases during periods of activity or stress and decreases during recovery and fasting phases. This teaches the body to utilize carbohydrates efficiently without dependence.

Fat metabolism represents the other side of metabolic flexibility. Efficient fat oxidation reduces inflammation, stabilizes energy, and supports long-term endurance. When fat oxidation pathways are suppressed by constant glucose availability, mitochondria become inefficient and oxidative stress rises. Reintroducing fat metabolism through fasting, low-glycemic meals, and overnight fasting windows restores mitochondrial balance. Longevity does not require permanent ketosis. It requires the ability to enter and exit fat-burning states smoothly.

Protein intake influences metabolic flexibility in subtle ways. High protein meals stimulate insulin modestly while activating growth pathways. Lower protein intake during fasting or rest phases allows insulin to remain low and fat oxidation to dominate. Protein cycling complements metabolic flexibility by aligning growth signals with feeding periods and repair signals with fasting periods. This balance prevents the chronic activation that accelerates aging while preserving lean tissue.

Circadian rhythm alignment further enhances metabolic switching. Insulin sensitivity peaks earlier in the day and declines in the evening. Eating late disrupts glucose control and fat oxidation simultaneously. Front-loading calories supports efficient fuel utilization, while extended overnight fasting restores metabolic rest. Longevity nutrition integrates timing with macronutrient selection, reinforcing natural biological rhythms rather than overriding them.

Stress undermines metabolic flexibility more than any macronutrient imbalance. Elevated cortisol increases glucose production, impairs insulin sensitivity, and suppresses fat oxidation. Under stress, even optimal nutrition can produce dysfunction. Longevity strategies must include nervous system regulation alongside dietary shifts. Metabolic flexibility emerges in environments of safety, not constant threat. When stress is reduced, the body regains the capacity to switch states without resistance.

Ultimately, metabolic flexibility is not about dietary identity. It is about adaptability. A long-lived organism is not optimized for one metabolic state but trained to move between many. Nutrition provides the training stimulus. By introducing intentional variability—fasting and feeding, carbohydrates and fats, protein abundance and restraint—the body relearns how to respond instead of resist. This responsiveness is one of the clearest markers of biological youth.

This chapter establishes metabolic flexibility as a prerequisite for all longevity nutrition strategies. Without it, fasting becomes stress, carbohydrate restriction becomes fatigue, and protein intake becomes inflammation. With it, nutrition becomes a dynamic system that restores resilience, stabilizes energy, and slows aging at its root.

The Day Her Energy Stopped Crashing

Maria had lived with energy swings for so long that she thought they were normal. Mornings were sharp but fragile. Afternoons collapsed without warning. Evenings were wired and restless. She ate frequently to prevent crashes, believing hunger was dangerous. Despite clean eating and consistent workouts, fatigue followed her like a shadow. Doctors labeled it stress. Nutrition plans labeled it noncompliance. Maria labeled it frustration.

What Maria didn't realize was that her body had lost the ability to switch fuels. Every snack kept insulin elevated. Every meal reinforced glucose dependence. Fat stores were locked away, inaccessible. Her mitochondria never rested. Energy crashes weren't failures of willpower—they were symptoms of metabolic rigidity. The change began quietly. Maria stopped snacking between meals. Not dramatically. Just enough to let insulin fall. At first, hunger felt alarming. Then it softened. She extended her overnight fast slightly and noticed her mornings became steadier. No crash. No urgency. Energy arrived calmly.

Next came carbohydrate cycling. Instead of eliminating carbs, she ate them intentionally after activity and earlier in the day. On rest days, meals leaned toward fats and proteins. Her body responded with something she hadn't felt in years: stability. Energy no longer spiked and crashed. It flowed.

As weeks passed, Maria noticed deeper changes. Her sleep improved. Cravings diminished. Mental clarity sharpened. Fasting days no longer felt stressful—they felt restorative. Her body began switching between fuels effortlessly, like a dimmer switch instead of an on-off button.

The most profound moment came during a stressful workweek. Normally, stress would unravel her routines. This time, her energy held. Her body adapted instead of collapsing. She realized flexibility was resilience. Her metabolism no longer panicked when conditions changed.

Maria stopped identifying as someone with “bad energy.” She understood her body had simply been trained incorrectly. By reintroducing contrast—feeding and fasting, carbohydrates and fats—she taught it how to respond again. Aging no longer felt inevitable. It felt negotiable.

Her story reflects a truth many never discover: longevity is not about finding the perfect diet. It is about restoring the body’s ability to adapt. When metabolism becomes flexible, energy stabilizes, inflammation recedes, and aging slows quietly in the background.

Metabolic flexibility didn’t make Maria superhuman. It made her human again. And in that return, youth quietly followed.

Chapter 3

Advanced Fasting Windows: Timing Autophagy Without Breaking the System

Fasting is often presented as a blunt instrument: eat less, wait longer, endure hunger, and reap benefits. This oversimplification has done more harm than good. In longevity science, fasting is not a test of willpower but a **precision tool** designed to activate specific biological repair processes at specific times. The goal of advanced fasting is not maximum deprivation, but **maximum signaling efficiency**. When fasting is applied intelligently, autophagy increases, insulin sensitivity improves, inflammation declines, and mitochondrial efficiency rises. When applied incorrectly, fasting elevates cortisol, suppresses thyroid function, accelerates muscle loss, and destabilizes hormones. Longevity fasting exists in the space between extremes.

Autophagy is the central mechanism through which fasting slows aging. It is the process by which cells identify damaged components, dysfunctional mitochondria, and misfolded proteins, then dismantle and recycle them. Autophagy is not binary. It exists on a spectrum. Short fasting windows initiate mild cleanup. Longer fasting windows deepen repair. However, autophagy competes with stress responses. If fasting pushes the body into perceived threat, repair is deprioritized. The nervous system must perceive safety for autophagy to operate optimally.

The timing of fasting determines which systems are affected. Overnight fasting of twelve to fourteen hours primarily improves insulin sensitivity and circadian alignment. Extending fasting to sixteen hours increases fat oxidation and begins activating autophagy. Fasting beyond twenty-four hours deepens cellular recycling but also increases physiological stress. Longevity fasting uses **layered exposure**, gradually training the body to tolerate deeper repair states without triggering hormonal disruption. The body must learn fasting, not be shocked by it.

Context determines fasting success. Age, sex, hormonal status, metabolic health, and stress load all influence how fasting is interpreted. Younger individuals with robust mitochondrial function tolerate longer fasts more easily. Individuals under chronic stress or with thyroid dysfunction may require shorter, more frequent fasting windows. Longevity nutrition rejects universal fasting prescriptions. Instead, it teaches adaptive fasting aligned with biological capacity. Protein availability strongly influences fasting outcomes. Entering a fasting window with depleted amino acid reserves increases muscle breakdown and stress hormone release. Longevity fasting pairs fasting windows with **strategic refeeding**, ensuring that periods of repair are followed by periods of rebuilding. This sequencing preserves lean mass while still activating autophagy. Fasting without repletion accelerates aging by weakening structural resilience.

Micronutrient status also determines fasting safety. Magnesium, sodium, potassium, and trace minerals regulate nerve conduction, blood pressure, and mitochondrial function during fasting. Deficiencies amplify fatigue, dizziness, and stress responses. Longevity fasting is supported fasting, not nutrient deprivation masquerading as discipline. Adequate hydration and mineral balance allow the body to enter repair mode rather than survival mode.

The relationship between fasting and hormones is often misunderstood. Fasting reduces insulin and IGF-1, which supports longevity, but excessive fasting elevates cortisol and suppresses thyroid output. Women, in particular, are sensitive to prolonged caloric restriction due to reproductive hormone signaling. Longevity fasting respects hormonal feedback loops, adjusting frequency and duration rather than forcing consistency. The goal is rhythmic signaling, not chronic suppression. Circadian timing amplifies fasting benefits.

Fasting that extends into the night aligns with melatonin release and cellular repair cycles. Late-night eating interrupts autophagy even if total calories are low. Front-loaded eating combined with early fasting enhances growth hormone secretion and mitochondrial repair. Longevity fasting integrates **when** with **how long**, recognizing time as a biological variable.

Psychological perception influences physiological response. When fasting is experienced as punishment, stress hormones rise. When fasting is framed as recovery, repair dominates. Longevity fasting includes cognitive reframing. Hunger becomes a signal, not a threat. Stillness replaces urgency. The nervous system shifts from defense to restoration.

Advanced fasting is not a permanent state. It is a periodic intervention layered within a broader nutritional system. Longevity emerges from cycles: feeding and fasting, building and cleaning, stress and recovery. This chapter establishes fasting as one phase in a repeating biological rhythm rather than a lifestyle identity. When fasting is timed correctly, supported nutritionally, and contextualized biologically, it becomes one of the most powerful anti-aging tools available.

The Quiet Hours That Rebuilt Him

Ethan began fasting because he was tired of feeling inflamed, heavy, and older than his years. Like many, he started aggressively. Long fasts. Black coffee. Ignoring hunger. Pushing through fatigue. At first, the scale moved and inflammation dropped. Then everything stalled. Sleep worsened. Training suffered. Mood flattened. He believed the problem was lack of discipline.

What Ethan didn't realize was that his body was no longer repairing—it was defending. His fasting windows were too long, too frequent, and unsupported. Cortisol rose. Thyroid output dropped. Autophagy competed with stress and lost. His body wasn't cleaning itself; it was conserving energy.

The shift came when fasting stopped being about endurance and started being about timing. Ethan shortened his fasts. He ate earlier. He added minerals and focused on refeeding properly. Hunger softened. Energy stabilized. For the first time, fasting felt calm.

He noticed something unexpected during those quiet fasting hours. Mental clarity increased. His body felt lighter, not weaker. Training days felt stronger because recovery improved. The silence between meals became restorative rather than tense.

Over months, Ethan learned to listen. Stressful weeks meant shorter fasts. Calm weeks allowed deeper ones. Fasting became fluid, responsive, intelligent. His body stopped resisting and started cooperating.

Blood markers improved. Sleep deepened. Muscle returned. Inflammation faded. Aging slowed not because he fasted more, but because he fasted **better**.

The most profound change wasn't physical. It was trust. Ethan stopped forcing his biology. He worked with it. Fasting became a dialogue instead of a demand.

In the quiet hours between meals, his body remembered how to repair itself. And in that remembrance, youth quietly returned.

Chapter 4

Protein Cycling for Longevity: Building Without Accelerating Aging

Protein is the most paradoxical nutrient in longevity science. It is essential for life, structure, and resilience, yet when consumed incorrectly, it accelerates aging. Protein builds muscle, repairs tissue, supports immune defense, and preserves metabolic function. At the same time, protein activates growth pathways that, when chronically stimulated, shorten lifespan by increasing cellular wear, oxidative stress, and metabolic demand. Longevity nutrition does not seek to eliminate protein or elevate it indefinitely. It seeks to **cycle protein strategically**, allowing the body to alternate between phases of growth and phases of repair.

At the center of this paradox lies mTOR, the mechanistic target of rapamycin. mTOR is a master regulator of growth. When amino acids—particularly leucine—are abundant, mTOR signals cells to build, divide, and synthesize protein. This is beneficial during development, recovery, and strength maintenance. However, when mTOR remains chronically elevated, autophagy is suppressed, damaged cells accumulate, and aging accelerates. Longevity is not achieved by suppressing mTOR entirely, but by **turning it on and off rhythmically**.

Protein cycling allows this rhythm to emerge. During higher-protein phases, muscle tissue is preserved, bone density is supported, and metabolic rate remains robust. During lower-protein phases, growth signaling quiets, autophagy increases, insulin sensitivity improves, and cellular cleanup resumes. This oscillation mirrors ancestral eating patterns, where protein availability fluctuated based on environment, season, and activity. Constant protein abundance is a modern condition that biology did not evolve to handle indefinitely.

Age significantly alters protein needs. In early and mid-adulthood, sufficient protein intake protects against muscle loss and metabolic decline. In later adulthood, inadequate protein accelerates frailty and insulin resistance. However, excessive protein at any age maintains elevated growth signaling that competes with longevity pathways. Protein cycling allows individuals to meet structural needs without paying the long-term cost of constant stimulation. The body is given permission to build—and permission to rest.

Protein timing matters as much as quantity. Consuming protein earlier in the day aligns with circadian rhythms, supporting muscle protein synthesis when insulin sensitivity is higher. Concentrating protein around activity amplifies its anabolic benefit. Lower-protein evenings allow growth hormone and melatonin to rise, supporting overnight repair. Longevity nutrition integrates timing so that protein signals reinforce natural biological cycles rather than override them.

Protein quality also determines longevity impact. Highly processed protein sources increase inflammation and oxidative stress. Whole-food proteins provide amino acids alongside micronutrients, fats, and bioactive compounds that moderate metabolic load. Plant proteins, animal proteins, and marine proteins each carry distinct signaling profiles. Longevity nutrition favors diversity rather than exclusivity, allowing the body to benefit from multiple amino acid patterns without excess exposure to any single one.

Fasting and protein cycling are complementary strategies. Fasting periods naturally suppress protein intake, quieting mTOR and enhancing autophagy. Refeeding periods reintroduce protein to rebuild tissue and restore strength. This sequencing protects lean mass while preserving repair capacity. Longevity is compromised when protein is restricted without repletion or elevated without restraint. Cycling creates balance.

Resistance training interacts powerfully with protein signaling. Exercise sensitizes muscle tissue to amino acids, allowing lower total protein intake to produce the same anabolic effect. This reduces the need for chronic high protein consumption. Longevity nutrition pairs training with targeted protein exposure, achieving strength preservation without persistent growth signaling.

Hormonal health further shapes protein tolerance. Thyroid hormones, insulin, and sex hormones influence how protein is utilized. Under chronic stress or hormonal imbalance, protein may increase inflammation rather than repair. Longevity strategies adjust protein intake in response to internal conditions rather than adhering to static targets.

Protein cycling ultimately reframes nutrition as **phase-based rather than fixed**. There are times to build and times to clean. Times to grow and times to conserve. By alternating these phases intentionally, the body avoids the trap of constant acceleration. Aging slows not because growth stops, but because it becomes purposeful.

This chapter establishes protein cycling as a cornerstone of the Longevity Nutrition Blueprint. When protein is used intelligently, it strengthens the body without aging it prematurely. When used carelessly, it accelerates decline. The difference lies not in grams, but in timing, rhythm, and respect for biology.

Stronger at Sixty Than at Forty

When Marcus turned sixty, he expected weakness to arrive quietly. He had spent decades lifting weights, prioritizing protein, and staying disciplined. Yet despite his efforts, joint pain increased, recovery slowed, and blood markers suggested rising inflammation. He ate more protein to compensate, believing muscle loss was the enemy. Instead, he felt heavier, stiffer, and more fatigued.

Marcus didn't know that his body was no longer asking for constant building. It was asking for balance. Every high-protein meal kept growth pathways active without allowing cleanup. His muscles were strong, but his cells were crowded with damage.

The change began with a counterintuitive suggestion: eat less protein—sometimes. Marcus resisted at first. Protein was his armor. But he experimented cautiously. On rest days, he reduced protein intake. On training days, he ate intentionally and early. He fasted lightly between cycles.

Weeks passed. His joints softened. Sleep improved. Training felt lighter, not weaker. His strength remained, but inflammation faded. Blood work improved without weight loss being the goal. Over time, Marcus felt something unexpected: resilience. His body adapted more quickly. Recovery accelerated. He realized that strength was no longer about pushing harder, but about alternating wisely.

At sixty-two, Marcus lifted with better form, fewer injuries, and more energy than he had at forty-five. Protein no longer ruled him. It served him.

He learned that longevity was not about denying growth, but about **earning it**. By allowing periods of restraint, growth regained meaning. Aging slowed not because he stopped building muscle, but because he stopped forcing it.

Marcus stopped fearing loss and started trusting rhythm. In that rhythm, his body found youth again—not as appearance, but as capacity.

Chapter 5

Micronutrient Precision: Feeding the Enzymes That Control Aging

Longevity is often framed in terms of calories, macronutrients, and fasting cycles, yet beneath these visible layers lies a deeper determinant of aging: micronutrient sufficiency. Vitamins, minerals, and trace elements do not provide energy, yet they enable every energy-producing reaction in the body. They act as cofactors, catalysts, stabilizers, and structural regulators for thousands of enzymatic processes that govern mitochondrial output, DNA repair, antioxidant defense, hormone synthesis, immune resilience, and detoxification. When micronutrient availability declines, these systems falter silently long before symptoms appear. Aging accelerates not because the body lacks calories, but because it lacks the molecular tools required to maintain itself.

Every cell relies on enzymes to function. Enzymes rely on micronutrients to operate. Magnesium stabilizes ATP and supports over three hundred enzymatic reactions. Zinc regulates gene expression and immune signaling. Selenium protects mitochondria from oxidative damage through glutathione peroxidase. Copper supports collagen cross-linking and antioxidant enzymes. Iodine enables thyroid hormone synthesis, which regulates metabolic rate and mitochondrial activity. B vitamins drive methylation, neurotransmitter production, and cellular replication. Without adequate micronutrients, biological repair slows while damage accumulates. Longevity depends on enzyme efficiency, and enzyme efficiency depends on micronutrient sufficiency.

Modern diets frequently provide sufficient calories yet inadequate micronutrients. Soil depletion, food processing, limited dietary diversity, and chronic stress all reduce nutrient density and absorption. Even individuals consuming whole foods may develop insufficiencies if intake lacks variety or if physiological demand increases. Stress, inflammation, environmental toxins, and intense training elevate micronutrient requirements. Longevity nutrition recognizes that requirements are dynamic rather than fixed. Nutrient needs shift with age, activity, hormonal status, and metabolic load.

Absorption is as critical as intake. Digestive function determines how effectively micronutrients enter circulation. Low stomach acid impairs mineral absorption. Gut inflammation disrupts transport. Imbalanced microbiota alter vitamin synthesis. Chronic stress reduces digestive enzyme output. Longevity nutrition therefore supports digestion alongside intake. Nutrients must be bioavailable, not merely consumed. Fermented foods, digestive support, and meal timing all influence absorption efficiency and thus longevity outcomes.

Micronutrient balance matters as much as quantity. Nutrients interact synergistically and competitively. Excess zinc depletes copper. High calcium impairs magnesium balance. Iron overload increases oxidative stress. Fat-soluble vitamins require adequate fats for absorption and proper ratios for safety. Longevity nutrition avoids megadosing and instead seeks equilibrium. The goal is sufficiency across systems rather than elevation of isolated nutrients. Balanced micronutrient status allows enzymatic networks to function harmoniously rather than unevenly.

Mitochondrial health is particularly sensitive to micronutrient status. The electron transport chain depends on iron, copper, B vitamins, magnesium, and coenzyme Q-related pathways. Deficiencies reduce ATP production and increase oxidative leakage, accelerating cellular aging. Antioxidant enzymes such as superoxide dismutase and glutathione peroxidase require zinc, copper, and selenium. Without these cofactors, oxidative stress rises even if caloric intake is optimal. Longevity nutrition therefore treats micronutrients as mitochondrial regulators rather than supplemental extras. Hormonal systems also rely on micronutrients. Thyroid hormones require iodine and selenium. Sex hormone synthesis depends on zinc and cholesterol metabolism. Adrenal function utilizes vitamin C and B vitamins. Deficiencies distort hormonal signaling, altering metabolism, mood, and repair capacity. Longevity nutrition stabilizes endocrine systems through micronutrient adequacy, allowing hormonal rhythms to support rather than disrupt aging processes.

The immune system similarly depends on micronutrients to distinguish threat from self. Zinc regulates immune cell maturation. Vitamin D modulates inflammatory signaling. Selenium supports antiviral defense. Deficiencies create chronic low-grade inflammation, a primary driver of aging known as inflammaging. Longevity nutrition reduces inflammatory load not only through macronutrient composition but through micronutrient sufficiency that allows immune regulation to function correctly.

Seasonality once ensured micronutrient variation. Different foods across seasons exposed humans to changing nutrient profiles, preventing chronic excess or deficiency. Modern diets eliminate this variability, leading to repetitive exposure patterns. Longevity nutrition restores diversity intentionally. Rotating vegetables, proteins, and mineral sources provides broader micronutrient coverage and reduces dependency on supplementation alone. Food diversity becomes a biological insurance policy against hidden insufficiencies.

Supplementation plays a supportive but secondary role. Supplements cannot replicate the complex matrix of whole foods, yet they can correct deficiencies when targeted precisely. Longevity supplementation prioritizes correction rather than accumulation. Biomarker-guided intake, moderate dosing, and periodic reassessment prevent imbalance. The aim is restoring enzymatic function, not achieving supraphysiological levels.

Micronutrient precision ultimately reframes nutrition from macronutrient management to biochemical support. Longevity depends on countless microscopic reactions occurring every second. When micronutrients are sufficient, these reactions proceed smoothly, repair exceeds damage, and aging slows quietly. When they are lacking, systems degrade despite caloric adequacy. Longevity nutrition therefore feeds not only the body's energy demands but its enzymatic intelligence.

The Missing Pieces She Couldn't See

Elena believed she was doing everything right. Her meals were clean, balanced, and disciplined. She exercised, slept well, and maintained a healthy weight. Yet fatigue lingered, hair thinned, nails weakened, and recovery slowed. Doctors found nothing alarming. "Normal aging," they said. Elena accepted the explanation reluctantly, assuming decline was inevitable.

What Elena couldn't see were the missing molecular pieces beneath her routines. Her food provided calories and macronutrients, but her diet lacked diversity. Magnesium intake was low. Selenium minimal. Zinc inconsistent. Iodine nearly absent. Her enzymes strained silently, working with incomplete tools. Energy production faltered not from lack of fuel, but from lack of catalysts.

The shift began subtly. Elena expanded food variety—seafood, seeds, mineral-rich greens, fermented foods. She corrected deficiencies gradually rather than dramatically. Meals became colorful, diverse, and seasonal. Nothing extreme. Just complete.

Weeks passed. Energy stabilized. Hair strengthened. Nails thickened. Sleep deepened. Training recovery improved. She felt restored in ways she hadn't expected. Aging seemed less aggressive, less certain.

Months later, blood markers reflected what she felt. Thyroid function improved. Inflammation declined. Antioxidant capacity rose. Elena realized her body had never been failing. It had been under-supplied.

The most profound change was perspective. She stopped viewing nutrition as restriction and began seeing it as provision. Food became a source of molecular support rather than calorie control.. Longevity felt less like resistance against time and more like cooperation with biology.

Elena learned that aging often accelerates not from visible neglect but from invisible absence. By restoring micronutrient completeness, she restored enzymatic harmony. Her body regained the capacity to maintain itself.

She did not become younger overnight. She became sustainable. And in sustainability, youth lingered longer.

Chapter 6

Nutrient Density & Food Diversity: Designing a Longevity Plate

Longevity nutrition is not built on restriction alone. It is built on density. While caloric excess accelerates aging, caloric sufficiency without micronutrient density produces a different but equally damaging outcome: biological undernourishment masked by fullness. A longevity plate is not defined by how little it contains, but by how much biological value it delivers per calorie. Nutrient density determines whether cells receive the materials required to repair DNA, maintain mitochondrial output, regulate hormones, and neutralize oxidative stress. Calories sustain survival. Density sustains longevity.

Nutrient density refers to the concentration of vitamins, minerals, phytonutrients, essential fats, amino acids, and bioactive compounds relative to caloric load. Highly processed foods provide energy but minimal enzymatic support. Even moderately healthy diets can fall short if food variety is narrow. Longevity demands a plate that supplies structural proteins, anti-inflammatory fats, antioxidant compounds, mineral diversity, and fiber for microbial health. Every meal becomes an opportunity to either deposit biological currency or withdraw from reserves.

Food diversity functions as biological insurance. Each plant and animal food carries unique micronutrient and phytonutrient profiles. Leafy greens provide magnesium and folate. Cruciferous vegetables support detoxification pathways. Berries deliver polyphenols that reduce oxidative stress. Fatty fish supply omega-3 fatty acids that lower inflammation. Seeds offer trace minerals essential for enzymatic balance. A repetitive diet narrows nutrient exposure and increases the likelihood of insufficiencies. Longevity nutrition intentionally rotates food categories to broaden nutrient coverage across weeks and seasons.

Phytonutrients deserve special emphasis in longevity science. These plant compounds, including flavonoids, carotenoids, glucosinolates, and resveratrol-like molecules, activate cellular defense pathways such as Nrf2. They increase endogenous antioxidant production rather than acting solely as antioxidants themselves. This distinction matters. Longevity is supported not by suppressing oxidative stress entirely, but by training the body to defend itself. Phytonutrient exposure provides mild hormetic stress that enhances resilience without overwhelming the system.

Fiber represents another underappreciated longevity nutrient. Beyond digestion, fiber feeds the gut microbiome, producing short-chain fatty acids such as butyrate that reduce inflammation and improve insulin sensitivity. The microbiome influences immune function, neurotransmitter production, and metabolic flexibility. A nutrient-dense longevity plate includes diverse fiber sources from vegetables, legumes, seeds, and resistant starches. Microbial diversity mirrors dietary diversity. When fiber variety declines, microbial ecosystems narrow, reducing resilience and increasing inflammatory tone.

Color diversity on the plate often reflects nutrient diversity. Deep greens signal chlorophyll and magnesium. Reds and purples indicate anthocyanins. Oranges suggest beta-carotene and carotenoids. Whites such as garlic and onions provide sulfur compounds essential for detoxification. Longevity nutrition encourages visual variety not as aesthetic preference but as biochemical strategy. A monotone plate rarely delivers comprehensive nutrient coverage.

Animal foods also contribute uniquely to nutrient density. Organ meats supply bioavailable B vitamins and trace minerals. Shellfish provide zinc and copper in balanced ratios. Eggs deliver choline for cellular membrane integrity. Fermented dairy or plant foods contribute probiotics that enhance absorption and immune modulation. Longevity nutrition does not adhere to ideological exclusion but evaluates foods by biological contribution. Seasonality once guaranteed diversity and cyclical exposure to nutrients.

Modern supply chains allow year-round availability but often at the cost of local density and freshness. Incorporating seasonal foods increases nutrient variability and encourages metabolic adaptation. Slight fluctuations in macronutrient and micronutrient intake prevent metabolic stagnation and maintain enzymatic responsiveness.

Overreliance on supplementation can inadvertently reduce dietary diversity. Supplements address deficiencies but do not replace the complex matrix of whole foods. Whole foods contain synergistic compounds that enhance absorption and regulate impact. Longevity nutrition prioritizes food-first diversity and uses supplementation as strategic correction rather than foundation.

Designing a longevity plate therefore involves structural layering. Protein for tissue maintenance. Healthy fats for membrane integrity and anti-inflammatory signaling. Diverse vegetables and fruits for micronutrients and phytonutrients. Fermented or fiber-rich foods for microbiome health. Periodic carbohydrate adjustments for metabolic flexibility. No single meal achieves perfection, but repeated density across days creates biological abundance.

Ultimately, nutrient density reduces the need for constant caloric excess. When cells receive adequate micronutrients, appetite regulation stabilizes. Cravings diminish. Energy stabilizes. The body stops seeking calories to compensate for micronutrient gaps. Longevity emerges not from deprivation, but from sufficiency delivered intelligently.

This chapter establishes the longevity plate as dynamic, colorful, and rotational. Diversity prevents stagnation. Density prevents deficiency. Together, they create a nutritional environment where repair exceeds breakdown and resilience replaces fragility.

The Plate That Changed Her Future

Sophia never felt malnourished. She ate regularly, avoided obvious junk food, and maintained a healthy weight. Yet she experienced subtle decline. Recovery after workouts lagged. Skin lost elasticity. Mood fluctuated. She dismissed these changes as normal aging.

One afternoon, reviewing her meals, Sophia noticed repetition. Oatmeal every morning. Chicken and rice most lunches. Salad with the same vegetables nightly. It was healthy, but narrow. Her body was fueled, but not enriched.

She began introducing variety deliberately. Different greens each week. Seafood twice weekly. Seeds rotated. Berries of different colors. Fermented vegetables added slowly. Meals became vibrant, layered, and textured. Nothing extreme. Just broader.

Within months, she felt different. Skin brightened. Energy steadied. Digestion improved. Cravings softened. Her body responded not to fewer calories, but to more completeness.

The most surprising shift was psychological. Eating felt expansive rather than restrictive. Meals became creative rather than calculated. She felt nourished at a cellular level she hadn't recognized before.

At her next medical check, inflammatory markers had declined. Lipid profiles improved. She hadn't lost weight intentionally, but body composition shifted subtly. Aging no longer felt like silent erosion. It felt manageable.

Sophia realized she had been surviving on adequacy rather than thriving on density. By broadening her plate, she broadened her resilience. Longevity didn't require heroic measures. It required completeness.

Her plate became a symbol—not of discipline, but of intelligence. Each color carried purpose. Each rotation restored balance. Aging slowed quietly, not through force, but through nourishment. Sophia stopped fearing time. She began feeding her future deliberately. And with each diverse meal, she built a body prepared not just to live longer, but to live well.

Chapter 7

Carbohydrate Cycling for Longevity: Fueling Performance Without Accelerating Aging

Carbohydrates occupy one of the most misunderstood positions in longevity nutrition. They are often portrayed either as essential fuel or as metabolic threat, yet neither extreme reflects biological reality. Carbohydrates are neither inherently aging nor inherently protective. Their impact depends entirely on context, timing, quantity, and metabolic state. In longevity physiology, carbohydrates function as signaling molecules that influence insulin, thyroid activity, mitochondrial respiration, and nervous system regulation. When delivered chronically and excessively, they accelerate metabolic aging. When applied cyclically and strategically, they enhance resilience, hormonal stability, and metabolic flexibility. Longevity nutrition therefore does not eliminate carbohydrates; it orchestrates them.

Insulin is the central mediator of carbohydrate signaling. Elevated insulin promotes glucose uptake and energy storage while suppressing fat oxidation and autophagy. Chronic insulin elevation leads to insulin resistance, inflammation, and mitochondrial stress—key drivers of accelerated aging. However, insulin also performs protective roles when activated appropriately. It supports anabolic repair, thyroid hormone conversion, and glycogen replenishment. Longevity depends not on suppressing insulin completely, but on allowing it to rise and fall rhythmically. Carbohydrate cycling restores this rhythm by alternating higher and lower carbohydrate exposure across time.

Metabolic flexibility determines carbohydrate tolerance. Individuals with robust insulin sensitivity and mitochondrial function utilize carbohydrates efficiently and clear glucose rapidly. Those with metabolic rigidity experience prolonged glucose elevation and inflammatory signaling. Longevity nutrition uses carbohydrate cycling to rebuild tolerance rather than eliminate carbohydrates permanently. Lower-carbohydrate phases enhance fat oxidation and insulin sensitivity. Higher-carbohydrate phases restore glycogen and support thyroid and nervous system balance. This oscillation trains the body to utilize both fuels without dependence.

Thyroid physiology is closely tied to carbohydrate availability. Adequate carbohydrate intake supports conversion of thyroxine to triiodothyronine, the active thyroid hormone regulating metabolic rate and mitochondrial output. Chronic carbohydrate restriction can suppress thyroid signaling, reducing energy expenditure and repair capacity. Longevity nutrition therefore includes periodic carbohydrate refeeding to maintain endocrine stability. Thyroid health is preserved not through constant carbohydrate abundance, but through strategic reintroduction.

The nervous system also interprets carbohydrate intake as a safety signal. Glucose availability reduces cortisol and supports serotonin production, influencing mood and sleep. Prolonged carbohydrate deprivation elevates stress hormones and disrupts circadian rhythms. Longevity requires balancing metabolic challenge with nervous system security. Carbohydrate cycling provides periods of metabolic rest that prevent chronic stress activation while still preserving insulin sensitivity.

Timing of carbohydrate intake profoundly alters its impact. Insulin sensitivity peaks earlier in the day and declines toward evening. Carbohydrate consumption aligned with activity or daylight enhances utilization and reduces storage. Late-night carbohydrate intake disrupts circadian biology, impairing glucose regulation and increasing fat storage. Longevity nutrition aligns carbohydrate exposure with circadian rhythms and energy demand rather than distributing it uniformly.

Activity level determines carbohydrate need. Physical exertion depletes glycogen and increases insulin sensitivity, making carbohydrates beneficial for recovery and performance. Sedentary periods reduce demand and favor lower carbohydrate intake. Longevity nutrition integrates activity-responsive carbohydrate availability, allowing fuel to match expenditure rather than exceeding it chronically. This alignment prevents both deficiency and overload.

Food quality further shapes carbohydrate signaling. Whole-food carbohydrates containing fiber, micronutrients, and phytonutrients produce slower glucose release and lower inflammatory response. Refined carbohydrates create rapid spikes and oxidative stress. Longevity carbohydrate cycling emphasizes nutrient-dense sources such as fruits, root vegetables, legumes, and intact grains while minimizing processed sugars. The goal is stable glucose exposure rather than volatile peaks.

Carbohydrate cycling ultimately mirrors ancestral patterns of feast and scarcity. Seasonal variation, activity-driven demand, and intermittent abundance prevented chronic insulin elevation. Modern diets flatten these cycles into constant availability. Longevity nutrition restores contrast intentionally. Periods of lower carbohydrate intake enhance fat metabolism and autophagy. Periods of higher intake replenish glycogen and stabilize endocrine systems. This rhythmic exposure preserves both metabolic efficiency and hormonal resilience. Longevity is compromised at both extremes: chronic high carbohydrate intake accelerates aging through insulin resistance, while chronic low intake impairs thyroid and nervous system function. Cycling resolves this tension by allowing carbohydrates to serve performance and recovery without driving metabolic deterioration. Aging slows when insulin signaling becomes dynamic rather than constant.

This chapter establishes carbohydrate cycling as a critical component of the Longevity Nutrition Blueprint. When carbohydrates are timed and varied intelligently, they support energy, mood, and metabolic adaptability. When consumed indiscriminately or suppressed entirely, they disrupt the very systems required for long-term health. Longevity nutrition therefore integrates carbohydrates as rhythmic signals rather than fixed macronutrient quotas.

The Fear of Carbs That Faded

For nearly a decade, Daniel avoided carbohydrates with quiet determination. Bread disappeared first, then fruit, then grains, then even starchy vegetables. He believed he was protecting himself from aging, insulin resistance, and weight gain. At first, results seemed promising. Weight dropped, energy sharpened, and discipline felt empowering. Over time, something shifted. Sleep became restless. Training felt heavier. Mood flattened. He ignored the signals, convinced restriction equaled longevity. Daniel's metabolism had adapted to scarcity but lost flexibility. Glycogen stores remained chronically low. Thyroid output declined subtly. Cortisol rose to maintain glucose supply. His body survived, but it no longer thrived. He mistook endurance for health.

The turning point came during a particularly exhausting month. Work stress increased, workouts stalled, and fatigue deepened. A coach suggested something Daniel resisted: reintroduce carbohydrates strategically. Not freely, not excessively—rhythmically. Higher intake after intense training. Lower intake on rest days. Earlier timing. Whole-food sources only.

Daniel approached cautiously. The first reintroduction felt unsettling. Fruit after training. Sweet potatoes with dinner on activity days. Nothing extreme. Yet something unexpected occurred. Sleep deepened. Muscles refilled. Energy stabilized. The constant edge of tension softened.

Weeks passed. He noticed warmth returning to his hands and feet, a subtle marker of metabolic health. Mood lifted. Workouts regained strength. Body composition remained stable. Carbohydrates had not undone his progress; they restored balance.

Months later, Daniel recognized the deeper lesson. He had not been harmed by carbohydrates. He had been harmed by rigidity. His body needed contrast, not exclusion. By alternating intake, he regained metabolic flexibility lost through chronic restriction.

The fear dissolved gradually. Carbohydrates became tools rather than threats. Some days abundant, other days minimal, always intentional. Aging no longer felt like a force to fight, but a process to guide.

Daniel's transformation was not dramatic. It was stabilizing. Energy flowed without spikes. Mood steadied. Recovery improved. He felt metabolically younger not because he avoided fuel, but because he used it wisely.

He learned that longevity did not require eliminating entire macronutrients. It required restoring rhythm. In that rhythm, his body remembered how to adapt—and adaptation is youth.

Chapter 8

Circadian Nutrition: Aligning Meals With the Body's Longevity Clock

Longevity is governed not only by what and how much is eaten, but by when nourishment occurs. Human physiology follows circadian rhythms—internal biological cycles synchronized to light, darkness, and activity. These rhythms regulate hormone release, metabolism, cellular repair, mitochondrial efficiency, immune function, and gene expression. Nutrition that aligns with circadian timing amplifies repair and metabolic efficiency. Nutrition that conflicts with circadian biology disrupts these systems, accelerating aging regardless of dietary quality. Circadian nutrition therefore represents one of the most powerful yet overlooked longevity strategies.

Insulin sensitivity follows a daily rhythm, peaking during daylight hours and declining in the evening. When carbohydrates and calories are consumed earlier in the day, glucose is cleared efficiently, and energy is directed toward activity and repair. Late-day eating produces prolonged glucose elevation, increased fat storage, and oxidative stress. Over time, this misalignment promotes insulin resistance and inflammation. Longevity nutrition aligns caloric intake with the window of highest metabolic readiness rather than distributing food evenly across waking hours.

Digestive physiology also follows circadian patterns. Gastric acid production, enzyme secretion, and gut motility are stronger during daytime activity and reduced during nighttime rest. Late-night meals therefore experience impaired digestion, reduced nutrient absorption, and altered microbiome interactions. Undigested substrates reaching the colon promote dysbiosis and inflammatory signaling. Circadian-aligned eating enhances assimilation and microbial balance, supporting longevity through improved nutrient utilization.

Melatonin, the hormone governing sleep and cellular repair, rises in darkness and is suppressed by food intake. Eating during the biological night blunts melatonin release, disrupting sleep architecture and mitochondrial restoration. Growth hormone secretion, which peaks during early sleep cycles, is similarly impaired by late feeding. Longevity depends heavily on nocturnal repair processes; circadian nutrition protects this window by creating fasting intervals before sleep onset.

Mitochondrial function fluctuates across the day in response to circadian gene expression. During active phases, mitochondria favor energy production. During rest phases, they shift toward maintenance and biogenesis. Eating late forces mitochondria into energy mode during a scheduled repair phase, reducing efficiency and increasing oxidative leakage. Over years, this mismatch contributes to accelerated cellular aging. Aligning meals with active periods preserves mitochondrial rhythm and longevity.

Peripheral clocks exist within organs such as the liver, pancreas, gut, and muscle. These clocks synchronize metabolic pathways to anticipated feeding times. Irregular eating patterns desynchronize these clocks from the central brain clock, producing metabolic confusion. The liver may expect fasting while nutrients arrive, impairing glucose regulation. The pancreas may anticipate feeding at times when no food arrives, disrupting insulin rhythms. Circadian nutrition restores predictability, allowing organ systems to coordinate efficiently.

Meal timing consistency strengthens circadian alignment. Regular eating windows train metabolic enzymes, hormone release patterns, and microbial cycles. Erratic timing produces hormonal variability and metabolic inefficiency. Longevity nutrition emphasizes stable daily feeding windows paired with overnight fasting periods long enough to permit repair. This consistency acts as a metabolic anchor, reducing physiological noise and stabilizing energy.

Shift work, late-night exposure to artificial light, and irregular schedules disrupt circadian biology profoundly. Individuals in such environments exhibit higher rates of metabolic disease, inflammation, and accelerated aging. Circadian nutrition becomes particularly protective under these conditions by preserving feeding-fasting cycles even when sleep schedules vary. Timing remains a modifiable longevity lever even in challenging environments.

Chrononutrition also interacts with fasting and macronutrient cycling. Fasting aligned with nighttime enhances autophagy and growth hormone release. Protein earlier in the day supports muscle synthesis when anabolic signaling is strongest. Carbohydrates earlier stabilize glucose regulation and serotonin pathways. Lower evening intake reduces insulin and preserves melatonin release. Longevity nutrition integrates macronutrient selection with circadian timing to amplify biological efficiency.

Psychological rhythms also align with circadian eating. Earlier meals promote stable energy and mood. Late eating correlates with impulsivity, cravings, and disrupted satiety signaling. Behavioral alignment supports adherence to longevity patterns without excessive effort. Circadian nutrition thus enhances both physiology and behavior simultaneously.

Ultimately, circadian nutrition reframes eating as a temporal event rather than merely a nutritional one. Food becomes a signal not only of nutrient availability but of time itself. When meals occur in harmony with internal clocks, metabolic pathways synchronize, repair processes dominate, and aging slows. When meals conflict with circadian biology, systems desynchronize and deterioration accelerates.

This chapter establishes meal timing as a foundational dimension of longevity nutrition. Even optimal foods lose protective effect when mistimed, while moderate foods gain benefit when aligned with biological rhythms. Longevity therefore depends not only on composition and quantity, but on temporal harmony with the body's internal clock.

The Evening Habit That Aged Him

For most of his adult life, Thomas believed his diet was healthy. He exercised regularly, avoided processed foods, and maintained stable weight. Yet sleep felt shallow, mornings sluggish, and inflammation markers crept upward each year. He attributed these changes to age and workload.

His days followed a predictable pattern. Breakfast was rushed or skipped. Lunch modest. Dinner large and late, often after long work hours. Evening meals became relaxation, reward, and routine. He fell asleep shortly afterward, believing a full stomach promoted rest. Thomas never considered timing as a biological factor. Food quality dominated his thinking. Yet his body experienced nightly disruption. Insulin remained elevated as melatonin attempted to rise. Digestion competed with repair. Growth hormone release diminished. Sleep cycles fragmented subtly. Night after night, repair windows shortened.

The realization came unexpectedly during travel. In a different time zone, he ate earlier by necessity. Dinner occurred before sunset. He slept deeper than he had in years. Morning energy returned. The shift felt disproportionate to such a small change.

Curious, Thomas experimented. He moved his largest meal earlier and reduced evening intake. Nights grew quieter internally. Sleep deepened. Morning clarity sharpened. Within weeks, energy stabilized throughout the day.

Months passed. Inflammation markers declined. Weight distribution shifted slightly toward lean mass. Mood steadied.

He had not changed foods dramatically—only timing. Longevity improved not through restriction but alignment.

Thomas recognized how long he had unknowingly worked against his biology. Late meals had quietly eroded nightly repair. By restoring circadian harmony, he restored restoration itself. The evening habit that once aged him became the anchor of his recovery. Meals earlier, nights quieter, mornings stronger. Aging no longer felt relentless. It felt negotiable. Thomas learned that longevity often hides in overlooked patterns. Timing, not just content, determines outcome. By respecting his internal clock, he reclaimed rhythms his body had waited years to express.

Chapter 9

Weekly & Seasonal Nutrition Cycles: Reintroducing Biological Contrast Across Time

Longevity does not emerge from static nutritional patterns. Biological systems evolved under conditions of fluctuation—periods of abundance and scarcity, variation in macronutrient exposure, seasonal shifts in micronutrients, and alternating metabolic demands. Modern diets have flattened these oscillations into constant availability, constant composition, and constant timing. While consistency offers predictability, excessive nutritional sameness produces metabolic stagnation. Cells adapt not to constancy, but to contrast. Weekly and seasonal nutrition cycling reintroduces this contrast intentionally, restoring metabolic responsiveness and slowing aging processes that arise from chronic uniformity.

Weekly nutrition cycles operate by varying macronutrient distribution, caloric load, and fasting duration across days. Periods of higher intake support anabolic repair, glycogen restoration, and hormonal stability. Periods of reduced intake enhance autophagy, insulin sensitivity, and mitochondrial efficiency. This oscillation mirrors natural patterns of exertion and recovery, allowing the body to experience both building and cleaning phases within short biological windows. Without these cycles, either growth pathways remain chronically activated or repair pathways remain insufficiently stimulated. Longevity depends on alternating both.

Protein cycling, carbohydrate cycling, and fasting windows become more effective when embedded in weekly rhythm. Higher protein and carbohydrate exposure aligned with training or activity days supports tissue repair and metabolic robustness. Lower protein and carbohydrate days quiet mTOR and insulin signaling, enhancing cellular cleanup. Fasting windows deepen on recovery days and shorten on anabolic days. Weekly cycling therefore integrates the mechanisms described in earlier chapters into a coherent temporal structure that sustains both strength and repair.

Seasonal nutrition cycles extend this principle across longer biological intervals. Historically, winter reduced carbohydrate availability and caloric intake, increasing fat oxidation and autophagy. Spring introduced plant diversity and micronutrient renewal. Summer increased carbohydrate exposure through fruits and activity. Autumn restored caloric abundance and protein intake before scarcity. These environmental rhythms trained metabolic flexibility and prevented chronic overexposure to any single nutrient pattern. Modern food systems eliminate these seasonal shifts, promoting continuous abundance. Longevity nutrition restores them deliberately.

Seasonal carbohydrate variation can enhance metabolic resilience. Periods of lower carbohydrate intake mimic scarcity, improving insulin sensitivity and fat metabolism. Periods of higher intake restore glycogen and support thyroid function. Similarly, seasonal protein emphasis can alternate between maintenance and repair phases. Micronutrient diversity naturally increases with seasonal produce rotation, reducing risk of deficiency or imbalance. These cyclical exposures maintain enzymatic adaptability and metabolic balance.

Psychological and behavioral benefits also arise from cyclic nutrition. Rigid dietary constancy often produces fatigue, monotony, and eventual nonadherence. Planned variation reduces psychological strain while maintaining biological benefit. Individuals experience abundance phases without guilt and restriction phases without deprivation because both are integrated into rhythm. Longevity nutrition therefore supports sustainability as well as physiology.

Metabolic memory develops through repeated cycles. When the body experiences predictable oscillations, enzymes regulating fat oxidation, glucose uptake, and mitochondrial biogenesis remain responsive. Constant intake patterns downregulate adaptability. Cycles preserve responsiveness across decades, maintaining metabolic youth. Aging often reflects loss of adaptability more than loss of capacity. Cyclic nutrition addresses this root cause directly.

Hormonal systems also benefit from rhythmic exposure. Thyroid signaling responds to carbohydrate availability. Sex hormones respond to energy sufficiency. Growth hormone responds to fasting intervals. Weekly and seasonal variation prevents chronic suppression or overstimulation of these axes. Endocrine balance emerges not from constant intake but from dynamic equilibrium across time.

Environmental alignment strengthens these effects. Increased activity in warmer seasons pairs naturally with higher carbohydrate tolerance. Reduced daylight and activity in colder seasons favor lower intake and deeper fasting. Aligning nutrition with environmental cues synchronizes circadian and metabolic rhythms simultaneously. Longevity nutrition thus becomes ecological as well as physiological.

Importantly, cyclic nutrition does not imply extreme

fluctuation or deprivation. The magnitude of variation remains moderate and supportive. The goal is contrast, not shock. Small shifts repeated consistently across weeks and seasons accumulate into meaningful biological signaling. Longevity emerges from sustained rhythmic exposure rather than occasional dramatic intervention.

Weekly and seasonal nutrition cycles therefore represent an advanced layer of the Longevity Nutrition Blueprint. By embedding fasting, macronutrient variation, and nutrient diversity into temporal structure, the body regains adaptive intelligence lost under constant conditions. Repair alternates with growth. Scarcity alternates with abundance. Responsiveness replaces rigidity. Aging slows because biology once again experiences the contrasts it evolved to interpret.

The Year Her Body Remembered

For most of her adult life, Hannah ate the same way every day. Breakfast identical. Lunch predictable. Dinner consistent. Her diet was balanced and disciplined, yet her energy plateaued, body composition stagnated, and motivation faded. She believed stability equaled health. Variation felt risky.

Years passed without obvious decline, yet vitality dulled quietly. Workouts produced fewer gains. Recovery slowed.

Mood flattened. Nothing dramatic—just gradual erosion. She blamed age.

A nutrition coach suggested something unexpected: change nothing dramatically—just introduce rhythm. Higher intake on active days. Lower intake on rest days. Seasonal rotation of foods. Slight fasting variation weekly. No extremes. Only contrast.

Hannah resisted at first. Predictability felt safe. Yet curiosity prevailed. She increased carbohydrates and protein on training days and reduced them gently on recovery days. She rotated produce with seasons instead of relying on the same staples year-round. Fasting windows lengthened slightly in winter and shortened in summer. The shifts were subtle, almost invisible.

Months passed before she noticed change. Energy stabilized. Training response improved. Body composition shifted gradually toward lean mass. Cravings diminished. She felt metabolically awake again, as if her body had re-engaged with its environment.

By the end of the year, Hannah realized the deeper transformation. Her body had remembered adaptability. Seasonal foods felt natural. Weekly variation felt effortless.

Eating regained vitality rather than monotony. Aging no longer felt like a fixed trajectory.

Medical markers reflected her experience. Insulin sensitivity improved. Inflammatory markers declined. Hormonal balance stabilized. No extreme diet had produced this shift. Rhythm had. Hannah understood she had not been failing before. She had simply been static. Biology had adapted to sameness and lost responsiveness. By restoring contrast, she restored youthfulness at a cellular level.

Her nutrition became a calendar rather than a template. Weeks breathed. Seasons rotated. Her body moved with time instead of against it. Longevity became experiential rather than theoretical.

She no longer feared aging as an unstoppable drift. She saw it as a process influenced by rhythm. And in reintroducing that rhythm, her body rediscovered resilience it had quietly waited to express.

Chapter 10

Integrating the Longevity Nutrition System: Designing a Lifelong Blueprint

Longevity nutrition reaches maturity when individual strategies become an integrated system rather than isolated practices. Fasting, protein cycling, carbohydrate variation, micronutrient density, circadian alignment, and weekly or seasonal rhythms each influence aging independently, yet their true power emerges only when synchronized. Human biology does not operate in compartments; metabolic, hormonal, mitochondrial, and circadian systems function as a network. Nutrition that supports longevity must therefore operate as a coordinated pattern across time rather than a collection of techniques applied sporadically. Integration transforms knowledge into physiology.

The first principle of integration is rhythm layering. Daily cycles govern circadian timing and overnight fasting. Weekly cycles alternate anabolic and repair phases. Seasonal cycles vary macronutrients and food diversity. These layers operate simultaneously, creating nested patterns of biological signaling. A day may include circadian-aligned meals. A week may include variable fasting windows and macronutrient distribution. A season may emphasize different foods and metabolic states. When layered coherently, these rhythms reinforce rather than conflict, amplifying longevity signaling across multiple timescales.

Metabolic flexibility acts as the foundation enabling integration. Without the ability to shift between fuels and states, cycling strategies become stressors rather than benefits. Integrated nutrition therefore begins with restoring flexibility through moderate fasting, macronutrient variation, and circadian alignment. Once flexibility is established, deeper cycles can be introduced safely. Integration respects sequence: adaptability precedes intensity. Longevity emerges when the body responds fluidly to variation rather than resisting it.

Protein, carbohydrate, and fasting cycles form the central metabolic triad of integration. Feeding phases emphasize protein and carbohydrate availability to support tissue maintenance, glycogen restoration, and endocrine stability. Repair phases reduce protein and carbohydrate exposure while extending fasting windows to enhance autophagy and fat oxidation. These alternating phases prevent chronic mTOR activation and chronic insulin elevation simultaneously. Integration ensures neither growth nor repair dominates indefinitely. Balance replaces excess. Micronutrient density and food diversity provide biochemical continuity across cycles. Regardless of macronutrient emphasis or fasting duration, meals remain nutrient-rich and diverse. This continuity ensures enzymatic function persists even as caloric or macronutrient exposure fluctuates. Integration therefore distinguishes between macronutrient cycling and micronutrient stability. Macronutrients vary to signal metabolic states. Micronutrients remain consistently sufficient to sustain cellular repair. This distinction prevents deficiency during variation.

Circadian alignment anchors all integrated cycles within daily time structure. Feeding occurs during metabolic readiness. Fasting extends into sleep phases. Macronutrient distribution aligns with activity and hormonal rhythms. Without circadian anchoring, weekly or seasonal cycles lose coherence. Integration therefore begins with time before composition. When meals occur at biologically appropriate times, metabolic pathways synchronize automatically. Temporal order precedes nutritional detail.

Psychological sustainability determines whether integration persists across decades. Longevity nutrition cannot depend on constant vigilance or extreme restriction. Integration allows flexibility within structure. High-demand periods can shift cycles temporarily without collapse. Social meals fit within feeding windows. Seasonal abundance phases permit enjoyment without guilt because repair phases follow naturally. Integration transforms longevity nutrition from discipline into lifestyle rhythm. Sustainability becomes inherent rather than forced.

Aging itself alters integration parameters. Younger individuals tolerate wider fasting variation and macronutrient extremes. Midlife requires increased protein cycling and circadian precision. Later life prioritizes anabolic support while maintaining mild repair cycles. Integration therefore evolves across lifespan stages. The blueprint adapts rather than remaining fixed. Longevity nutrition is dynamic architecture, not static prescription.

Biomarkers provide feedback for integration refinement. Energy stability, sleep quality, body composition, inflammatory markers, glucose regulation, and hormonal balance reflect nutritional harmony. Integration uses these signals to adjust cycle magnitude and timing. The body becomes both subject and guide. Longevity emerges when feedback informs pattern rather than forcing pattern despite feedback.

Environmental and lifestyle factors also integrate with nutrition. Physical activity increases carbohydrate and protein tolerance. Stress increases micronutrient demand and reduces fasting tolerance. Seasonal light exposure influences circadian rhythm and appetite. Integration considers context rather than isolating diet from life conditions. Nutrition becomes adaptive interface between organism and environment.

Ultimately, the Longevity Nutrition Blueprint is not a protocol but a system of relationships. Timing relates to hormones. Macronutrients relate to metabolic state. Micronutrients relate to enzymatic function. Cycles relate to adaptability. Integration harmonizes these relationships across time. Aging slows because biology experiences coherent signaling rather than conflicting inputs.

This final chapter establishes integration as the culmination of longevity nutrition. Individual strategies initiate improvement, but synchronized rhythms sustain it across decades. When daily, weekly, and seasonal cycles align with metabolic, circadian, and environmental realities, nutrition becomes a lifelong regenerative force. Longevity ceases to be a goal and becomes a pattern lived continuously.

The Pattern That Lasted

When Robert first began improving his health in his forties, he approached nutrition like a project. Diets came and went. Fasting phases alternated with high-protein phases. Carbohydrate restriction followed by reintroduction. Each strategy worked briefly, then faded. Results improved, then plateaued. He believed longevity required constant effort and vigilance.

Years passed in cycles of enthusiasm and fatigue. Progress never fully stabilized. He blamed inconsistency, assuming discipline was the missing piece. What he did not see was fragmentation. His strategies existed separately rather than as a unified pattern. His body received conflicting signals across days and seasons.

The shift began in his early fifties when he stopped chasing new methods and began observing rhythms. Energy peaked earlier in the day. Hunger varied across weeks. Winter appetite differed from summer. Training cycles influenced recovery needs. Instead of imposing rigid plans, he aligned nutrition with these patterns.

Meals moved earlier naturally. Fasting windows extended slightly overnight. Protein rose on active days and softened on rest days. Carbohydrates increased in warmer months with activity and declined in quieter seasons. Food diversity rotated with availability. Nothing extreme. Only coherence.

Months turned into years. Unlike previous attempts, the pattern persisted. Weight stabilized effortlessly. Energy remained steady. Sleep deepened. Medical markers improved gradually and stayed improved. Aging no longer felt adversarial. It felt guided. Robert realized he had stopped "doing" nutrition and started living it. Integration replaced effort. Cycles replaced rules. The body responded not because he forced change, but because he synchronized with it.

At sixty, he felt more capable than at forty-five. Not through intensity, but through continuity. Longevity emerged quietly from sustained alignment. The pattern lasted because it matched biology rather than overriding it.

Robert's experience reflected a simple truth: longevity does not come from perfect days. It comes from coherent years. When nutrition becomes rhythm instead of regimen, the body maintains itself naturally.

He no longer measured success in pounds or phases. He measured it in stability. And stability, sustained across time, became youth preserved.

Chapter 11

Adaptive Nutrition Across the Lifespan: Evolving Longevity From Youth to Late Life

Longevity nutrition is not static because human biology is not static. Nutritional needs, metabolic responses, hormonal environments, and repair capacity evolve continuously across the lifespan. Strategies that enhance resilience in youth may require modification in midlife and recalibration in later decades. The Longevity Nutrition Blueprint therefore extends beyond cycles and timing into adaptation across age-related physiological shifts. Aging is not a failure of nutrition but a change in nutritional interpretation. Adaptive nutrition recognizes that the same inputs produce different outputs as biological systems mature.

In early adulthood, metabolic flexibility and mitochondrial capacity are typically robust. Insulin sensitivity is high, anabolic signaling is efficient, and recovery processes operate with minimal intervention. Nutrition during this phase primarily reinforces resilience rather than restoring it. Moderate fasting, diverse nutrient exposure, and balanced macronutrient cycling maintain adaptability without excessive restriction. Excessive deprivation during youth can impair hormonal stability and long-term metabolic capacity. Longevity nutrition in early life therefore emphasizes sufficiency, diversity, and rhythmic variability rather than aggressive intervention.

Midlife introduces subtle metabolic shifts. Insulin sensitivity often declines, circadian rhythms weaken, and stress exposure accumulates. Mitochondrial efficiency decreases gradually, while inflammatory tone rises. Hormonal transitions—particularly in thyroid and sex hormones—alter nutrient utilization. During this phase, longevity nutrition becomes more deliberate. Circadian alignment grows more important. Fasting windows require precision rather than extension. Protein cycling gains relevance to preserve lean mass while still permitting repair. Carbohydrate timing becomes critical to maintain metabolic flexibility. Adaptation replaces assumption.

Later adulthood changes nutritional priorities further. Sarcopenia risk increases, digestive efficiency declines, and micronutrient absorption may weaken. Anabolic resistance emerges, meaning muscle protein synthesis responds less robustly to intake. Fasting tolerance may narrow due to reduced metabolic reserves. Longevity nutrition therefore shifts toward anabolic support balanced with gentle repair cycles. Protein intake often increases in frequency and quality, while fasting becomes shorter but still present. Nutrient density becomes paramount as caloric intake often declines. The goal transitions from optimization to preservation without accelerating aging.

Hormonal transitions across lifespan require adaptive macronutrient strategy. Declining estrogen or testosterone alters insulin sensitivity, fat distribution, and protein metabolism. Thyroid signaling may decrease with age, reducing metabolic rate and mitochondrial output. Longevity nutrition compensates by adjusting carbohydrate timing, protein distribution, and micronutrient sufficiency to support endocrine balance. Static dietary identities fail under changing hormonal conditions; adaptive nutrition evolves alongside them.

Digestive physiology also changes with age. Gastric acid production often declines, impairing mineral absorption and protein breakdown. Microbiome diversity may narrow with reduced dietary variety or medication exposure. Longevity nutrition responds with increased food diversity, fermented foods, and nutrient bioavailability emphasis. Protein sources may shift toward easier digestion, while mineral-rich foods and supportive digestion practices become more relevant. Nutrient assimilation becomes as important as intake.

Recovery capacity narrows with age due to mitochondrial decline and reduced repair signaling. Nutrition must therefore balance stress and restoration more carefully. Fasting intervals remain valuable but must avoid excessive catabolism. Carbohydrate cycling continues but emphasizes stable glucose regulation. Protein cycling favors preservation of lean tissue while maintaining intermittent repair phases. Adaptive nutrition maintains longevity signaling without exceeding physiological tolerance.

Psychological relationships with food also evolve across lifespan. Early rigidity often softens into intuitive patterns. Longevity nutrition encourages alignment with internal cues rather than imposed structures, particularly in later years. Sustainable rhythm replaces strict adherence. Adaptation acknowledges that longevity requires decades of continuity rather than periods of intensity. The most effective nutrition is the one that persists through life transitions.

Environmental and lifestyle factors further shape lifespan nutrition needs. Activity patterns change, stress exposures fluctuate, and social contexts evolve. Longevity nutrition adapts to these shifts rather than resisting them. Physical activity reductions require macronutrient recalibration. Increased stress requires micronutrient support and reduced fasting intensity. Adaptive nutrition remains responsive to context as much as age. The concept of metabolic age becomes more relevant than chronological age. Individuals of the same chronological age may exhibit vastly different metabolic flexibility, mitochondrial capacity, and hormonal balance. Longevity nutrition adapts to biological markers rather than calendar years. Feedback from energy stability, recovery capacity, body composition, and metabolic markers guides adjustments. Adaptation is personalized rather than generalized.

Ultimately, adaptive nutrition across the lifespan reframes longevity from prevention to stewardship. Early life builds resilience. Midlife maintains flexibility. Later life preserves capacity. The Longevity Nutrition Blueprint evolves continuously, respecting biological shifts while sustaining core rhythms. Aging slows not because change is resisted, but because nutrition changes with it intelligently.

This chapter establishes adaptive evolution as the final dimension of longevity nutrition. The blueprint does not end at maturity; it accompanies the organism across decades. When nutrition evolves alongside biology, longevity becomes not merely extension of years but preservation of function across them.

The Seasons of His Body

At twenty-five, Alex never thought about aging. He ate freely, trained intensely, and recovered easily. Energy returned overnight. Hunger guided him without effort. Nutrition felt simple: eat enough, move often, sleep when tired. His body adapted automatically.

By forty, things felt different. Recovery slowed. Fat accumulated subtly. Energy fluctuated. Alex responded as he always had—by pushing harder. Longer fasts. Lower carbohydrates. More training. Results came briefly, then fatigue deepened. He assumed discipline had faded.

What Alex did not recognize was that his body had changed seasons. Strategies that once enhanced resilience now exceeded tolerance. His metabolism no longer responded to force but to balance. Yet he treated his forty-year-old physiology as if it were twenty-five.

The turning point arrived after persistent fatigue forced reflection. Instead of intensifying restriction, he softened it. Fasting shortened slightly. Protein intake distributed across meals. Carbohydrates reintroduced around activity. Meals earlier. Diversity increased. Nothing radical—only responsive.

Within months, energy stabilized. Training improved. Sleep deepened. His body felt cooperative again. Alex realized he had not lost discipline; he had ignored adaptation. Longevity required evolution, not persistence in old patterns. Years later, at sixty, another transition emerged. Appetite declined. Muscle maintenance required intention. Fasting tolerance narrowed. Alex adapted again. Protein quality increased. Fasting became gentler. Nutrient density rose. Activity adjusted. His body responded with preservation rather than decline.

Alex came to see his life as nutritional seasons. Youth required abundance. Midlife required rhythm. Later years required protection. Each phase honored biology rather than resisted it. Longevity became continuity through change.

Looking back, he recognized the most powerful shift was perspective. Aging was not deterioration—it was transformation requiring adaptation. Nutrition that evolved allowed function to persist. He remained capable not because he fought age, but because he moved with it.

At seventy, Alex felt neither young nor old. He felt aligned. His body had carried him through decades because he learned to nourish each phase differently. Longevity was not frozen youth. It was sustained vitality across time.

The seasons of his body continued, but decline did not dominate them. Adaptation did. And in adaptation, life extended not only in years, but in capacity.

Epilogue

Longevity as a Living Rhythm

Longevity is often imagined as a destination, a point reached after enough discipline, enough knowledge, or enough control. Yet the deeper truth revealed throughout this book is that longevity is not something achieved once. It is something practiced continuously. It lives in rhythms rather than rules, in patterns rather than perfection. Nutrition, when aligned with biology, becomes not a diet to follow but a relationship to maintain across time.

The Longevity Nutrition Blueprint began with a shift in perception: food as signal rather than substance. From that foundation emerged the pillars of fasting, protein cycling, carbohydrate variation, micronutrient precision, nutrient density, circadian timing, and weekly and seasonal rhythm. Each principle revealed that the body is not static. It responds, adapts, remembers, and recalibrates. Aging accelerates when inputs remain constant and misaligned. Aging slows when inputs vary rhythmically and harmonize with internal systems.

What becomes clear at the end of this journey is that longevity nutrition does not require intensity. It requires coherence. The body thrives when signals across time reinforce one another. Meals earlier in the day protect circadian repair. Fasting windows restore cellular cleanup. Protein cycles preserve tissue without chronic growth activation. Carbohydrate rhythm maintains metabolic flexibility. Micronutrient density sustains enzymatic intelligence. Seasonal variation restores ecological alignment. These are not separate interventions but interwoven strands of one living pattern.

Equally important is the realization that longevity nutrition evolves. Youth favors abundance and flexibility. Midlife favors rhythm and metabolic precision. Later years favor preservation and nutrient density. The blueprint is not rigid because biology is not rigid. Adaptation across life stages ensures that longevity is not confined to any single decade but carried forward continuously. Nutrition becomes stewardship of capacity rather than resistance to change.

Perhaps the most profound insight is psychological rather than biochemical. Longevity does not thrive under fear. Fear of hunger, fear of carbohydrates, fear of calories, fear of aging itself—these states elevate stress physiology that undermines repair. The Longevity Nutrition Blueprint replaces fear with understanding. Fasting becomes restoration rather than deprivation. Feeding becomes support rather than indulgence. Cycling becomes rhythm rather than restriction. The body responds differently when nourishment is cooperative rather than adversarial.

Longevity also emerges from sustainability. Extreme regimens rarely persist across decades. Rhythmic patterns do. When nutrition aligns with natural cycles of day, week, and season, adherence becomes effortless because behavior matches biology. Consistency arises not from willpower but from compatibility. The most effective longevity strategy is the one that can be lived indefinitely without strain.

Across this book, the theme of contrast reappears repeatedly. Feeding and fasting. Growth and repair. Abundance and restraint. Activity and rest. These contrasts are not opposites in conflict; they are partners in balance. Biological youth depends on experiencing both sides of each pair. Constant feeding ages. Constant fasting weakens. Constant protein accelerates. Constant restriction depletes. Longevity lives between extremes, in oscillation that preserves responsiveness.

The modern environment removed much of this contrast. Food became constant, seasons muted, activity optional, light artificial. The Longevity Nutrition Blueprint reintroduces contrast intentionally to restore what environment once provided naturally. This restoration is not regression to the past but alignment with biological design. Human physiology evolved for rhythm. When rhythm returns, resilience returns. As you close this book, the goal is not memorization of protocols but recognition of patterns. Longevity is sustained when meals align with daylight, fasting aligns with darkness, macronutrients vary with activity, micronutrients remain dense, and cycles unfold across weeks and seasons. These patterns are adaptable to any culture, cuisine, or lifestyle because they reflect universal biology rather than specific foods. The blueprint is flexible because its foundation is physiological rather than prescriptive.

There will be days of abundance and days of restraint. Weeks of high activity and weeks of rest. Seasons of metabolic challenge and seasons of nourishment. Longevity does not demand that these variations disappear. It requires that they integrate. When nutrition responds to life rather than resisting it, health persists across change. The body becomes resilient not through control but through alignment.

Longevity is therefore not an outcome secured at some future point. It is a living rhythm practiced daily. Each aligned meal, each appropriate fast, each nutrient-dense plate, each circadian-timed evening contributes a small signal toward repair. Over years, these signals accumulate into preserved function, stable energy, and sustained vitality. Aging slows not dramatically but steadily, as coherence replaces conflict.

The Longevity Nutrition Blueprint ultimately teaches that the body already knows how to maintain itself. What it requires is an environment of signals that permit it to do so. When nutrition provides that environment consistently across time, longevity ceases to be theoretical. It becomes lived experience. Not youth regained, but vitality extended. Not immortality pursued, but function preserved.

The rhythm continues beyond these pages. Each day offers another opportunity to reinforce it. And in that continuity, life lengthens not only in years, but in quality.

www.ingramcontent.com/pod-product-compliance
Lightning Source LLC
LaVergne TN
LVHW022016200926
848481LV00007B/2420